Art as Therapy

For Retirees

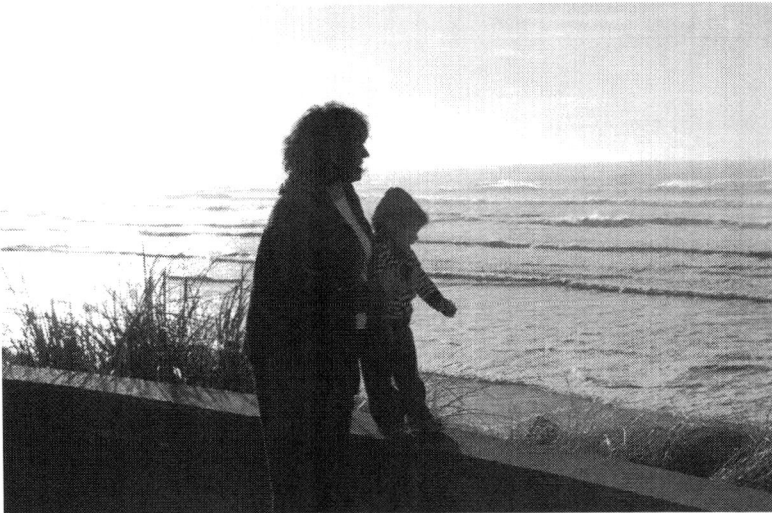

Written by Lola Carlile, Ph.D.

2012 copyright Masabi Press
PO Box 2663
Salem, OR 97308

For information, contact the author @
masabitherapist@gmail.com.

ISBN-13: 978-1481265379

ISBN-10: 1481265377

Carlile, Lola.
Art as Therapy for Retirees

Therapy, depression, art therapy, anxiety, stress, retirement, retirees

Contents

1. You knew it was coming. What did you expect?
2. Defining retirement
3. Keeping busy
4. Laughing
5. Scheduling
6. Learning
7. Keeping it Simple
8. Cursing
9. Exercising
10. Finances
11. Romance
12. Five Senses
13. Defying the Odds
14. Write Your Own Story
15. Don't Depend on Your Kids!

Appendix

Dedicated to all my friends who retired before me and those who will yet venture on to this new turf – retirement. May it be wondrous, fulfilling, and the highlight of

your life story!

Chapter 1
You Knew It Was Coming. What DID You Expect?

I'm not just retiring from the company; I'm also retiring from my stress, my commute, my alarm clock, and my iron. ~Hartman Jule

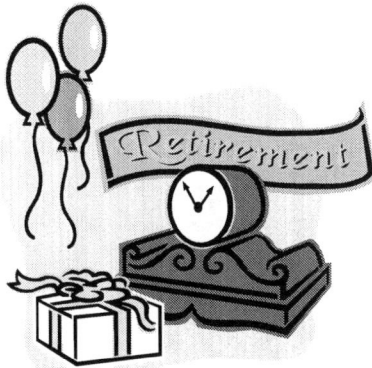

Year two in retirement. True retirement. When I retired the first time at age fifty-eight, I went to art therapy school. So I didn't really retire that time. But when I graduated from art therapy school, I actually did retire for a year or so. I didn't have a schedule. There were days I didn't get out of my nightgown. I didn't even brush my teeth and forgot to take my medicine. And I just slept a lot.

Therapists might say that I was lazy or depressed. I think it was a bit of both. I've always been very active, going, running, planning, and doing. All of a sudden no one cared. I didn't have to be anywhere. I didn't have to even wake up if I didn't want to.

If it weren't for having to use the restroom, I swear I could have slept all day long and then into the night, only to wake for a while to roll over and go back to sleep. Sometimes the dreams were so good I did not want to wake up.

And then something happened. I thought, "Is this all there is? Is this what I am doing? Just vegging out until I die?"

What are you looking forward to in retirement? What have you done that you have enjoyed? Draw them! Remember, this is an art therapy workbook. You gotta write in the pages. C'mon, you can do it....OK, if you are art challenged, draw simple stick figures OR write if you absolutely have to! Use the whole next page for your doodling!

So, whether you planned well for your retirement or just arrived there with no premeditated thought, this book is for you. Take it and work out the pieces either by yourself or with a group of friends. You might like the way you feel when you are finished!

Retirement does not have to be slowing down. You may find you are even more active and on the go more than you ever expected. It's just a matter of perspective and planning.

My friend Annie urged me to add something else to this book and that is to tell you why art might be as good or even a better format for you to think and learn new things about yourself. Well, this one thing has to do with my Bible Study class. As an admittedly lukewarm Catholic, I never took a Bible Study class until this past year. During one of the classes the leader invited us to journal our thoughts. Now, as a writer, I should be very compliant with that directive, correct? Wrong.

I did not want to write. I sat there and finally started doodling. I am not a natural born artist and drawing does not come easily to me, but I do make some dynamite flowers and I began to make my little curved lines and then sat looking at the flower.

My, my, I thought. *I wonder why plants always die at my house. Could it be that I forget to water them? Could it be that I don't care or even try to care for them? Hum...so, with this Bible study thing. . . . Am I going to really read this stuff at home and do worksheets? Something tells me no....*

And then it hit me – the art! Yes, the art stimulated my brain to think in a way just writing did not. Amazing. So, art helped me reframe my thoughts so I could journal. As if I really did at that time....uh, nooooo!!!
So, go on and try to draw or use some magazine pictures when asked to do something. You don't have to do anything if you don't want to. But then I ask why are you reading this book if you don't wanna somehow try and cooperate? ☺

The second illustration I will give you is my darling mama. She wondered why in the heck I returned to graduate school to study anything remotely to do with art. In her words: "We don't do art. None of us do."

So, I sat down with my mom and handed her a pencil and a sheet of paper and said, "Draw!"

Of course she commented about not being able to draw and I simply said, "Just scribble then."

And, yes, she did. She gripped the pencil in her hand so hard I thought it might disintegrate and she clenched her jaw and began drawing concentric circles almost breaking the point of the pencil.

Voila! There it is, Mom! I almost shouted to her- When we examined her "art," we both agreed that it represented her entire attack on life – do it hard, strong, and emotionally. Yep. The energizer bunny had nothing on my mom. And mom looked at me and said, "OH! I get it!"

The light bulb was on and she understood the power of art and her blessings were showered upon me for finding this niche in my life.

Draw what you think your life looked like before retirement. Describe it in 5 words!

My life was: (use five words to describe what was): Draw what your life is like now that you are retired or if you are contemplating life as a retiree soon....

Write!

_____

_____

_____

_____

_____

_____

_____

_____

_____

_____

Draw!

My life as a retiree now is: (use five or 50 words to describe what is):

Write!

_____

_____

_____

_____

_____

_____

_____

_____

_____

_____

Draw!

What is the difference between now and then?

Write!

_____

_____

_____

_____

_____

_____

_____

_____

_____

_____

_____

Imagine yourself relaxed, happy, and fulfilled. What does that place look like?

Write!

_____

_____

_____

_____

_____

_____

_____

_____

_____

_____

_____

_____

Draw some things that might be in that picture. Who is there? What things are there? What is the landscape like? Take a deep breath. Put on some cool and inspirational music and imagine you are THERE!

If you could think of one thing that might make you happier right now, what would that one thing be?

Write!

_____

_____

_____

_____

_____

_____

_____

_____

_____

_____

_____

_____

_____

_____

Draw!

This isn't an art class. No one is going to grade you and no one has to even see it. This is just for YOU!

Chapter 2
Define Retirement

I enjoy waking up and not having to go to work. So I do it three or four times a day. ~Gene Perret

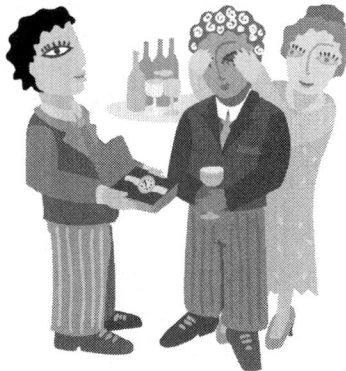

Retirement is defined newly as "changing, and that has caused a lot of confusion. Retirement used to be considered the end of things and the beginning of old age. Now, since we live longer and are healthier, more and more people see retirement as a great opportunity to do new things and find more meaning in their lives."
http://www.jackdwilliamsphd.com/aboutretirementcoaching/definingretirement.html

A lot of us prepare for new careers or work on our hobbies that we only had a bit of time for earlier in life. Others end up being the perennial babysitter for the grandkids. Whatever we are doing, it is not what our grandmothers and grandfathers were doing necessarily. Many of us have lots of energy and abilities that we want to utilize. And so we do….

We are currently a group of individuals who want to feel good about life and we want to make a difference. Man y of us are baby boomers and we were known for love in any season during the sixties and in the 2000's we want to be known and heard as those same hard-working, hard-playing folks who want to make life meaningful for those around us. We aren't the I generation. The generation that thinks of what can I get...but the one who wants to make sure that others get the best out of life.

Sometimes big changes occur when we retire. Sometimes those changes are limited to income, but other times, those include moving to another place, getting help with daily activities, losing one's autonomy, and medical problems.

What has changed for you? Think of how you felt, looked, and acted during your working days. Now think of how you are in the present. Close your eyes and visualize what was and what is. On the next two pages, get your funk on and start a drawing'....

What did you look like or how did you feel when you worked fulltime? Or when the kids were all at home and you multi-tasked day in and day out...

Write!

_____

_____

_____

_____

_____

_____

_____

_____

_____

_____

_____

_____

Draw!

Remember, this is for your eyes only. You can use just colors to represent how life was back then. Abstract is good!

Now think of how you feel and act. What colors represent how you might be today?

Write!

_____

_____

_____

_____

_____

_____

_____

_____

_____

_____

_____

Draw!

some lines or squiggly marks to indicate your life now. Again, abstract is good!!! Just scribble and enjoy yourself!

Think about what your ideal retirement would look like, with money being NO object! Enjoy this drawing. Allow yourself to dream big....Write first about what you might draw.

Write!

_____

_____

_____

_____

_____

_____

_____

_____

_____

_____

_____

_____

Draw!

Your ideal retirement life....

As you were drawing, did you think of other things? Like what?

Write!

_____

_____

_____

_____

_____

_____

_____

_____

_____

_____

_____

_____

_____

_____

Draw!

What did your grandparents' or parents' retirement look like?

Write!

_____

_____

_____

_____

_____

_____

_____

_____

_____

What are the major differences in your retirement and your grandparents or parents?

Write!

_____

_____

_____

_____

_____

_____

_____

_____

Draw!

Chapter 3
Keeping Busy

Rest is not idleness, and to lie sometimes on the grass under trees on a summer's day, listening to the murmur of the water, or watching the clouds float across the sky, is by no means a waste of time. ~J. Lubbock

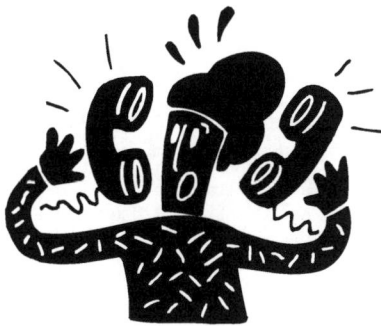

Just as Lubbock said, rest does not mean you aren't doing anything. What it really says to me is that rest means you are doing things that do not stress you out. You are resting or retiring from the demands of life that sometimes make you a little crazy or even a bit under the weather. You can take time to decide what to do and you are not under the gun having to decide in a hurry.

But let it not be said that you should stay in the house and/or yard and go nowhere. You must schedule your life, but not as hectically as young people seem to need to do!

When I was sleeping the days away, I found out that I just existed. So, now I try to schedule some things a few times a week. I have something to look forward to doing. A few ladies and I have formed a movie club, whereby on Friday afternoons we meet for lunch at the local Applebee's and then trek on down to our artsy and very comfortable local cinema and watch a movie. We read the reviews of the flick and then share our

thoughts as we munch on celery sticks and drink nonfat lattes (NOT)!
People are just plain social beings and even the most adroit and independent soul among us needs people contact sometimes. Another group I enjoy is our AAUW Cooking Group (as long as they don't discuss politics, 'cause these girls are way too liberal for me). We meet once a month at someone's home and they do all the cooking and serving and we just pay ten bucks to the hostess. Works for me....

You hear a lot of talk about volunteering. Well, don't volunteer unless what you are volunteering to do is a passion for you. I found that I do not like tutoring as much as I thought I would, even though I absolutely LOVED teaching. It's just not a part of my life now. What I enjoy more than anything is writing and sharing with people. So, writing this book is cathartic for me. What is your passion?

What might you like to do that you have never had time to do?

Write!

_____

_____

_____

_____

_____

_____

_____

_____

_____

_____

_____

_____

_____

Draw!

Draw several things that please you just to think about doing. Don't worry if they aren't practical. This is your time to dream....

What things would you really NEVER EVER want to do again?

Write!

_____

_____

_____

_____

_____

_____

_____

_____

_____

_____

Draw!

We're going to get real now! Just think of something that interests you, but you have no practical experience or know how of this particular thing.

What is it and why might you want to learn about it? What is your secret ambition?

Write!

_____

_____

_____

_____

_____

_____

_____

_____

_____

_____

_____

_____

Draw it and, guess what? You might want to take a class to learn about it. Ask someone who is an expert in the field, etc. My husband was interested in religions of the world so he took a series of classes, beginning with Islam. He loved reading about the religion, reading the Quran, and visiting a mosque. So, what's your secret ambition?

What are you good at?

Write!

_____

_____

_____

_____

_____

_____

_____

_____

_____

_____

_____

_____

What are some things you really are not good at? (To be honest, I was a horrible artist and almost didn't make it into art therapy school. I had to take extra classes in art, but if you check out the index, you will see some of my art – not bad for a non-artist!)

Write!

_____

_____

_____

_____

_____

_____

_____

_____

_____

_____

_____

Draw!

So, now pick one or two of your passions and make a goal sheet. What is your goal for the next month? Year? Five years? Use your strengths as your aid.

Write!

_____

_____

_____

_____

_____

_____

_____

_____

_____

_____

Draw!

Chapter 4
Laughing

According to a new survey, women say they feel more comfortable undressing in front of men than they do undressing in front of other women. They say that women are too judgmental, where, of course, men are just grateful. -Jay Leno

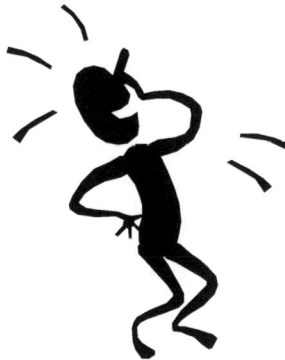

Let's be honest. When was the last time you laughed out loud? And when was the last time you laughed out loud and cried and couldn't stop? The last time I laughed out loud was when viewing an episode of "King of Queens." That show makes me laugh. I'm not sure, but it may be that my husband likes it and, therefore, I do as well. He laughs out loud and we have a great time talking about the shows that kind of remind us of ourselves. We also enjoy other sitcoms, such as "Everyone Loves Raymond." Yep, those are the upper shows that make life a bit more enjoyable.

What stars make us laugh? Joan Rivers and Don Rickles were two of our favorites because they said it like it was. They were pre-PC (politically correct) times.

Do you tell jokes? Do you read jokes? Do you laugh at yourself? Laughter heals. There is no way to avoid it. When we laugh we release pheromones that heal our bodies. So why aren't we laughing more?

Seinfeld makes me laugh. Just listen: **There's very little advice in men's magazines, because men don't think there's a lot they don't know. Women do. Women want to learn. Men think, "I know what I'm doing, just show me somebody naked." -Jerry Seinfeld**

When my granddaughter visits and tries to put on a mad face or start throwing a fit, I laugh out loud. Before you know it, she can't keep that "go to hell" expression on her face anymore. She joins me in laughter!

Once during my respite as a retiree, one of my sons said he wanted me to be his funny mom again instead of a whining, needy woman. Yeah, others want to be around us when we are fun. And, we don't have to have liquor to be funny. Or do we?

What do you need to be funny? What puts you in the mood?

What gets you in a LAUGHING MOOD?

Write!

_____

_____

_____

_____

_____

_____

_____

_____

_____

_____

Draw!

Okay, joke time! Write down at least two funny jokes. If you can't think of any, go to the internet, Google **HUMOR** and you'll get a plethora of ideas. Illustrate each one. Use two pages!

JOKE #1

Write!

_____

_____

_____

_____

_____

_____

_____

_____

_____

Draw!

JOKE #2

Write!

_____

_____

_____

_____

_____

_____

_____

_____

_____

_____

_____

_____

Draw!

What was the name of the last funny movie or television show you watched? What was funny about it?

Write!

_____

_____

_____

_____

_____

_____

_____

_____

Draw!

Recall the last funny thing that happened to you. Why it was funny. Can't think of a thing? Relax. Read a few jokes. Laugh. Smile. If you do it long enough, you will elevate your mood even if you have to force yourself at first.

Write!

_____

_____

_____

_____

_____

_____

_____

_____

_____

_____

Draw!

Chapter 5
Scheduling

The key is not to prioritize what's on your schedule, but to schedule your priorities.
Stephen Covey

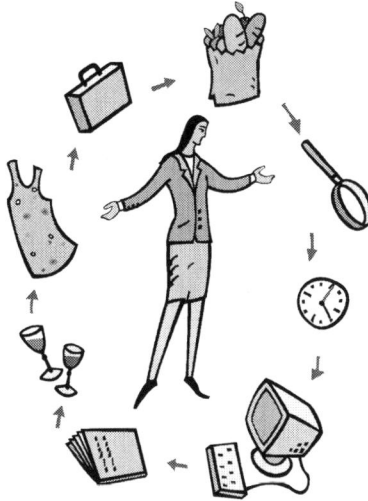

What are your priorities? I mean the things you have to do. Doctor appointments are important, as are birthdays and family celebrations. I can't recall the number of important things I have missed due to forgetting. We all forget, so we need to devise a way to remember things. Okay, I'm honest here: I bought so many calendars, having great intentions mind you, and lost them. So what works for me may not work for you.

Some people put a magnet on the fridge with the week's schedule. Not the fun stuff, but the have to do stuff! Others find that they are reasonably successful with a calendar on their desk. Some people use a computer's calendar and others put sticky notes on the bathroom mirror. Whatever works for you is great.

Don't forget your moral support group. Have someone remind you of an important date in the coming week. I've found it does not help to try to remember too much. Just the important stuff. Sometimes a luncheon engagement is very important as well.

I read about one hint I had not thought of but like very much: send yourself an email! Remind yourself.

One friend told me that she put a ribbon around her thumb and when she went to bed; she took it off and in the morning, put it on again. The week went by, but by the end of the week, she didn't remember what it was for and the appointment she was supposed to remember was long missed!

Sometimes we don't remember things because they just aren't that important to us. Yeah, going to the dentist is important. But I would just as soon forget about it, especially if I need some work done....Sometimes it's just convenient to forget.

Think about what helps you remember. On the next page, draw the ways you can remember to do things and do them on time!

I REMEMBER THINGS WHEN I.....What helps you to remember things?

Write!

_____

_____

_____

_____

_____

_____

_____

_____

_____

_____

_____

How does it feel when you remember things and arrive on time to occasions?

Important events for the next year: Write and draw something for each one. For example,

Hubby's Birthday

Draw!

Which of these events do you look forward to? Why?

Write!

_____

_____

_____

_____

_____

_____

_____

_____

_____

_____

_____

Draw!

Look at next week! What are you planning? Fill in the calendar below with quips, remarks, comments, and pictures!

Write and Draw!

Sun	Mon	Tue	Wed	Thu	Fri	Sat

Things to do while you are waiting for an appointment:

Write!

_____

_____

_____

_____

_____

Draw!

Doodle. Close your eyes. Take a pencil and move it. When you are finished, look at what you drew. Can you see anything in the doodle? Color it in!

Draw!

Chapter 6
Learning
The only good is knowledge and the only evil is ignorance.
Socrates

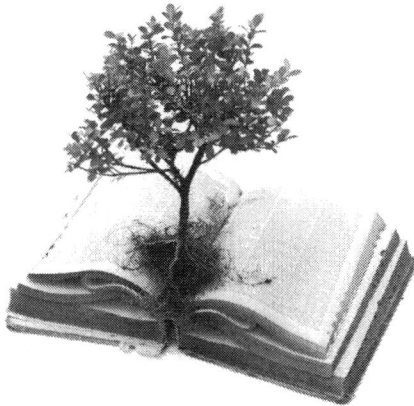

I am fortunate indeed, as my mother instilled in me a love of learning. I must admit it was not some altruistic belief of the wonder of learning that I learned, but the fact that I was not to be disturbed when I was reading. I didn't have to do dishes. I didn't have to do any work if I was reading. So, guess what? I read all the time. And there began my love of learning. I read fiction, nonfiction, and anything in between.

My family honored education and learning. I married a man who is intellectually curious as well. But there are people I know who don't read, who don't care about learning, and who are pretty well ensconced in non-educational pursuits. Well and good for all of them, but if pressed, they would admit they do read for information. They do read manuals to figure out how to fix their cars or look up on the Internet ways to order a certain something. We are continually learning even if we don't suspect it....

Now that you are retired, you will learn some things, like never leaving a candle burning while you are out of the house, or that you should leave your keys in the same place every time you come home...those kind of things are practical learning situations. But the ever growing dendrites in our brain expand and duplicate when we learn new things. For instance, do you know what synthesisia is? Well, some of society's members, albeit a small number, have this trait. It is when you see colors when you hear music. I mean you see the colors in your head! Cool, eh? When you learn something new that is interesting to you, your dendrites shake and roll and connect tighter and make more connections, enhancing your brain. This is a good thing!

Think of something new you might want to learn or somewhere new you might want to visit. What could you do to make that experience more meaningful? I once wanted to write a book for kids and families to enjoy countries by learning to speak a few phrases, eat some of the food, enjoy the music, and do some of the folk art. It's that kind of thing that makes us different from the animals, who do the eating, sleeping, walking, and talking (barking or meowing or whatever) bit. We can do much more and when we do, our brains thank us by working far more efficiently.

Ready? What do you want to learn about? If you can't think of a single thing, then think about something you love and then think of something you could learn about it. If you enjoy football, maybe you could learn about one of the players – his life story. If you love music, perhaps you could find a new CD out by one of your favorite artists. So, play with me – draw some things you want to learn more about....

Write!

_____

_____

_____

_____

_____

_____

Draw!

Are you active in your community? Do you make a difference? What are some things you could learn about your community that would make a difference to those who live there? It could even be the best place to eat.

Write!

_____

_____

_____

_____

_____

_____

_____

_____

_____

_____

Draw some things in your community below.

Why did you draw what you drew? Did you surprise yourself? Why or why not?

What new routes can you walk around your home? If it's raining, you can just walk around the house, looking at each piece of furniture in the house. Contemplate each piece. Why is it here?

Write!

_____

_____

_____

_____

_____

_____

_____

_____

_____

_____

Draw five things in your walk.

What one piece could you get rid of? To whom could you bestow it? Why did you think of that person? Your brain is working, friend! Keep it moving!

Write!

_____

_____

_____

_____

_____

_____

_____

_____

_____

_____

Draw!

Think of a place to go. Visit this URL:
http://www.50plusexpeditions.com/ 50plus
Expeditions

This is a senior only tour company. They offer tours all over the world but they specialize in North American tour packages for the senior citizen. Where would you want to go if you had carte blanche?

Write!

_____

_____

_____

_____

_____

_____

_____

_____

_____

_____

_____

_____

Draw a map of where you might want to go (create a place – it can have rivers, boats, fish, whatever you'd like.

What has to be in this picture? What one thing would you not want to do without?

Write!

_____

_____

_____

_____

_____

_____

_____

_____

_____

_____

_____

Draw!

Whether you have to pack for a vacation or a move, you need to think about what you need and want to take with you. How much can you get into one suitcase? Can you travel light?

Write!

_____

_____

_____

_____

_____

_____

_____

_____

_____

_____

Draw!

What do you know about your community? What are some of the places you could visit. Why would you go there? With whom would you go?

Write!

_____

_____

_____

_____

_____

_____

_____

_____

_____

_____

Draw!

Chapter 7
Keeping It Simple

Simplicity is the peak of civilization." – Jessie Sampter

Life is not complex. We are complex. Life is simple, and the simple thing is the right thing. Oscar Wilde

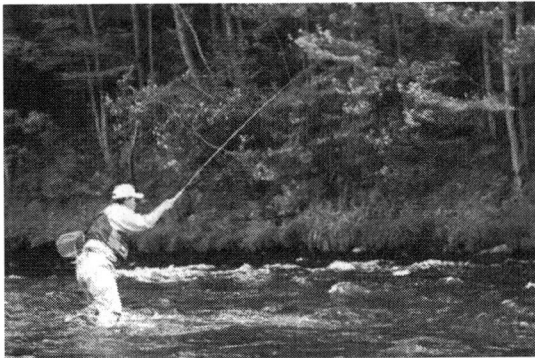

I remember the first time I heard the acronym PDQ (pretty damn quick). I was working in a pharmacy and everything was simplified. We had to work hard and fast. We wanted to please the clients. Our vocabulary was simplified. It worked. We did a good job.

The acronym for Keep it simple, stupid (KISS) became a mantra of teachers. We wanted to make sure we kept the kids in tune by keeping our explanations simple enough to do the job, but easy enough for the kids to learn. KISS was the mantra in writing class. Keep it simple! Note to lawyers and government agencies: KISS!

So life in retirement should be simple and fun. It should be simple enough so that we can enjoy our life. We can enjoy our families. And we can enjoy good health. Stress is the #1 health buster in the world. Cancer and all sorts of disease thrive on stress. So now that we know THAT, why don't we try to eliminate stress?

Begin by organizing your life better. You don't have to attend every birthday party under the sun, especially those of you with huge families.

If they stress you out, send a card, good wishes, and a promise to go out to lunch some day, just the two of you. Some people are stressed out by large groups. You do not have to go places where there are large gatherings. Your mother and/or father won't make you go. You just simply don't have to go.

The other day I was stressed out about some county precinct work committee I had applied for. It was for NO PAY, but they had interviews. I was so stressed out about the interview, I finally had to call them and tell them I could not come to the interview. Can you imagine being on that committee? Stress city was all I saw down the road. I could have avoided stress altogether by NOT applying for the position in the first place. Of course, I should place priorities in my life. That makes life simpler. My hubby was sick at the time and that was the confounding factor.

So, how can you simplify your life? Begin by your living arrangements. Yep. Look around you. If you are like the majority of us, you have a lot of stuff. Just like George Carlin said, "We buy bigger places so we can fill them with more stuff."

Pick out one room in your house or apartment. Check out all the things that are in there. Come back to the book. Name ten things in that room. *Do* you **NEED** all those things? Don't they complicate your life with having to be dusted and/or cleaned in some way?

Write!

_____

_____

_____

_____

_____

_____

_____

_____

_____

_____

Draw at least three items to get rid of in that room.
And then do it!

How do you feel about getting rid of these things? After giving them away, do you miss them? Probably not....

Simplify. Beautify. I could go into my head and do a lot of simplifying there. When certain things happen, I am the first to figure out a bunch of negative reasons why X happened. For instance, I apply for a job. I don't get an interview. I think it's because I'm old. I think it's because somehow they don't like me, although they have never met me. And so on....What's in your head that you could get rid of? Thoughts, thoughts, and then some more thoughts....Write them down and then rub them out! (Can erase, but I'd suggest drawing all over those negative thoughts really hard!) Get rid of clutter!

Write!

_____

_____

_____

_____

_____

_____

_____

Draw!

How does it feel to rub out some negative thinking?
Simplify your thinking.

Write!

_____

_____

_____

_____

_____

_____

_____

_____

Words of wisdom: It's a matter of perspective. If I want to feel good, I will think good thoughts. I will attribute all good things to what is going on and if someone else is rude, I'll just think, "Poor fella, he must be having a hard day" and say a prayer for him.
Modern day Pollyanna

Identify what is important to you. Get rid of everything else. Simplifying your life is not a task – it's a journey. Are you ready for it? What are some things you really love and with which you do not want to part?

Write!

_____

_____

_____

_____

_____

_____

Do you know why those things are so important to you? Really? Write the reason here.

Write!

_____

_____

_____

_____

_____

_____

_____

_____

_____

_____

Draw!

Look through your wardrobe. Do you have clothing you haven't worn in 20 years? We all do. Come on, admit it! Are these garments serving any purpose in your life? Tell what you are thinking about those unused garments....

Write!

_____

_____

_____

_____

_____

_____

_____

_____

_____

_____

Draw!

Is there a better place for them to be and why? You know the answer. Write it down. Read it aloud.

Write!

_____

_____

_____

_____

_____

_____

_____

_____

_____

_____

_____

Draw! Draw where they could or should be....

Another way to simplify your life is to "be in the moment." Enjoy the moment. Don't look back and don't look forwards. Just be there. Life is so much more enjoyable if you try it. Just think what you are doing right now.

Write!

_____

_____

_____

_____

_____

_____

_____

_____

_____

_____

Color in the shape below and just think about how calm you are, how beautiful the colors are and how great it is to be alive....

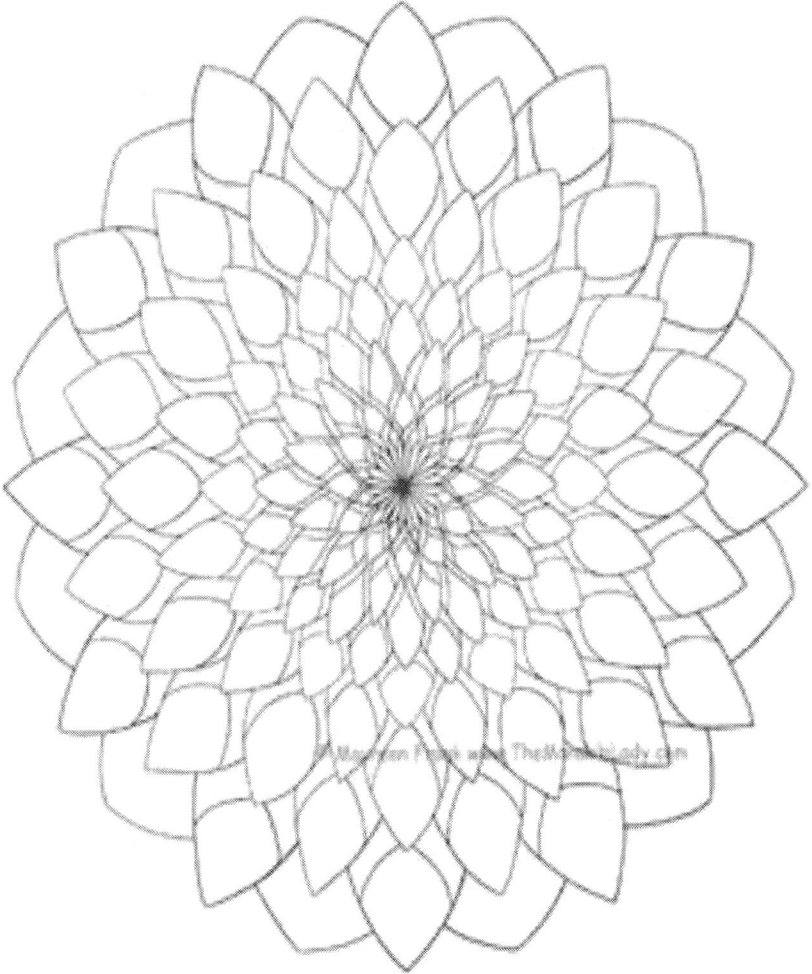

Chapter 8
Cursing

Cursing is invoking the assistance of a spirit to help you inflict suffering.

Swearing on the other hand, is invoking, only the witness of a spirit to a statement you wish to make.
John Ruskin

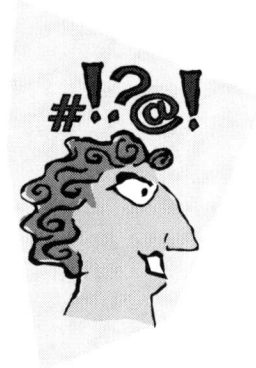

Cursing is a gift of the military, you might say, to me. My father was a sergeant in the army and I heard words I thought were German (-ck suffix which sounded pretty German to me) until I went to college. It came in handy not responding to cursing when I taught middle school. The kids could never irritate me, since I didn't really hear the bad words, hence they stopped the cursing! It's a modern miracle that I never used those words I was so used to hearing in school. I might not be talking about retirement now had I used them!

Geriatric Profanity Disorder, Also known as G.P.D.

A common medical disorder in which a cantankerous, old, senior citizen will not stop swearing. Usually directed toward ungrateful "youngsters" meaning anyone from 1 to 55 years of age. The reasons behind this ailment are quite simple. They've lived long enough that they no longer give a shit whom they annoy. So you damn well better listen, you ingrate, or you're gonna get a cane upside your head.

It is quite natural that there will come a day when you just get so mad you feel you could burst. Those who hold it in do damage; however, they don't immediately know it. But your organs take the beating! So what's the problem with cursing? It's better than physically injuring someone. It diffuses the moment especially if you misuse the adjectives. Using humor can dissipate anger and that's a good thing. Think of the words you cannot stand. Think of ones that are raunchy, but you might use them. My dear mother in law once said "damn" and I was shocked. My own mother would not say goddamn it, but she would say god darn it! So, however your vocabulary goes, know that once in a while it's okay to let off steam.

Scientists say something about the amygdala and cursing activating that when you swear especially when you're hurt — and they say it is a good thing! So, don't beat yourself up by letting one slip once in a while. It can be healthy!

Write!

My NO swear list:

Why are these words on this list?

Swear words to use when I really need to let it go!

Draw!

Scribble your heart away! When you get mad, just write, scribble, and tear up some paper! What works for you when you are mad?

Group Therapy

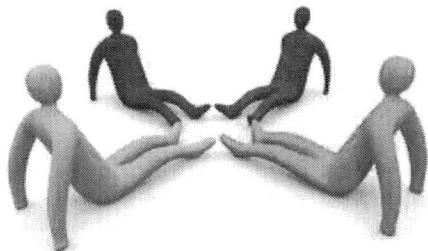

Write the names of people whom you can count on to help you out in a crisis or when you have problems....you might even say what it is about them that makes you feel safe in writing their name(s) here!

Write!

_____

_____

_____

_____

_____

_____

_____

How do you deal with anger? Close your eyes. Think of something that has made you angry. How did you feel? Your body? Your breathing? Draw the parts of you that react when you're stressed.

Draw!

Expressing Your Emotions (see the site address below for this)

At this point, take a deep breath and start to block out all outside noises and influences. The painter should tell themselves "I am here for *me*. I am not here to impress anyone and no one ever needs to see the end results, this time is about *me*."

This process is going to express emotions with paint and canvas; let the paint and the music move the painting. Start to feel the stress being relieved. With this process the painter will be able to express his anger, happiness, or whatever he is feeling.

To begin the process, use any brush and dip it into one of the colors of paint or dip half of it in one color and the other half in another color. Start to apply this to the canvas in any way that feels good. Brush it on with long slow strokes, dab it on with tiny little dabs or smear it on with a scrubbing motion – whatever suits the mood. Relax and let the emotions flow.

Take a deep breath and let it out. Take another brush, fill the brush with another color or colors and use a different technique than the first one. Paint in a different spot or over the last spot – it doesn't matter, just paint. Use the emotions to guide the hand. The painter should be able to close her eyes and feel the paint mixing with the canvas and to feel the stress leaving her body.

Alternate brushes and colors and strokes, use the music to set the speed of the strokes. Dab to the beat, stroke with the guitar rhythm or smoosh with the tuba, whatever is felt. Let go of any anger.

Take a deep breath and let it out. Use another brush, a rag, a sponge, hands or whatever else that can be thought up and do some more painting. Use a plastic spoon and scrape some of the paint off that was earlier applied, or grab a glass and swirl the lip edge around in the paint – let the imagination run wild. No need to worry about conventional thinking; think more about being a child. Remember finger painting!

Step back and look at what has been done. It's beautiful! Even if the eyes don't know it, the soul will understand the emotions and repression that was released and it will be beautiful.

Read more at Suite101: Art Therapy Painting for Stress-Relief: Learn to Paint Emotions and Feelings | Suite101.com http://suite101.com/article/art-

therapy-painting-for-stress-relief-
a128307#ixzz1xGJ2aaFH

Use your canvas to paint something beautiful! It doesn't have to look like anything. Just enjoy the colors!

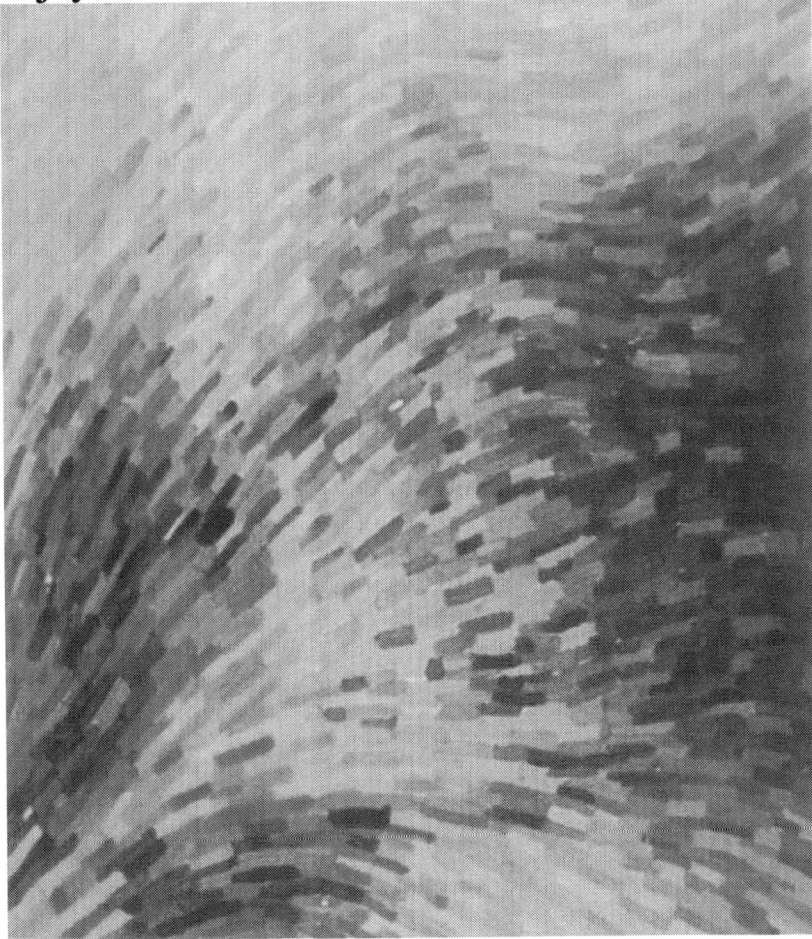

Look at your painting. What do you like about it? What would you change? How are you feeling now?

Write your thoughts on the next page!
Write!

_____

_____

_____

_____

_____

_____

_____

_____

_____

_____

_____

Draw!

Chapter 9
Exercising

Lack of activity destroys the good condition of every human being, while movement and methodical physical exercise save it and preserve it. *~Plato*

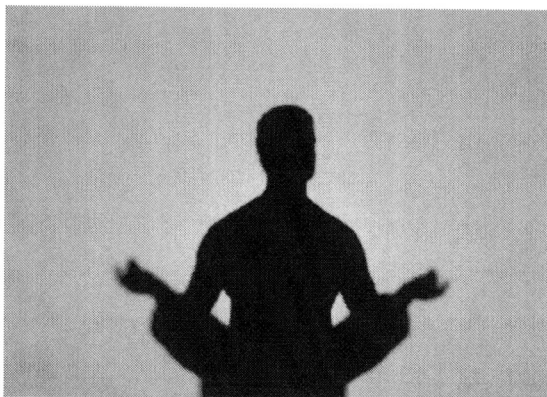

Now, how am I going to in good faith talk to you about exercising when it's the one thing I have always disliked? I am saddened to share with you that I don't like moving. I don't like starting to move. I read. I work on the internet. I write. I love those things. But do I love getting up and walking on the treadmill? NO. Absolutely not. But as we get older, we have to move or we will lose it. Seriously, lose it! Have you had days when you just sat around and slept all day? Is that living?

I have found one type of exercise I do like and that's water aerobics. I don't really enjoy going to the group things, so I go by myself and work out. I can't swim, but I can swim with a noodle to support me. That works great. And I feel so good when I am through. But I am lucky to go twice a week. It's getting myself there that is the big problem. Do you have that problem? If not, you are one up on all of us slackers.

Another relaxing and helpful movement is to walk a labyrinth. But if you don't know where your local labyrinth is, you can create your own! I started a path I walk in my home and I usually have some great music playing and I just relax and walk that route over and over again, sometimes for thirty minutes or so. It really helps clear the mind and activate the organs.

A lot of people call the labyrinth a spiritual journey. It doesn't have to be that, but anything involving the mind could be called spiritual, right? Take the next page and follow the labyrinth with your pencil. Relaxing, right? You cannot get lost in a labyrinth. These are ancient tools used for meditation and relaxation.

One exists at Marylhurst University where I studied to be an art therapist. I never knew what it was or why those lines were on the parking lot until my last semester at the school. I tried walking it several times and found it very relaxing and satisfying. You don't know until you try it....

Yoga, Pilates, and other wonderful classes await you, but you don't even have to do them anywhere but in the privacy of your own home. CDs are available to help you create the best life for you and that includes your mind, spirit, and body. Take care of them, 'cause no one else will. And, if you care to check it out, when you don't feel well physically, your emotional well being suffers as well.

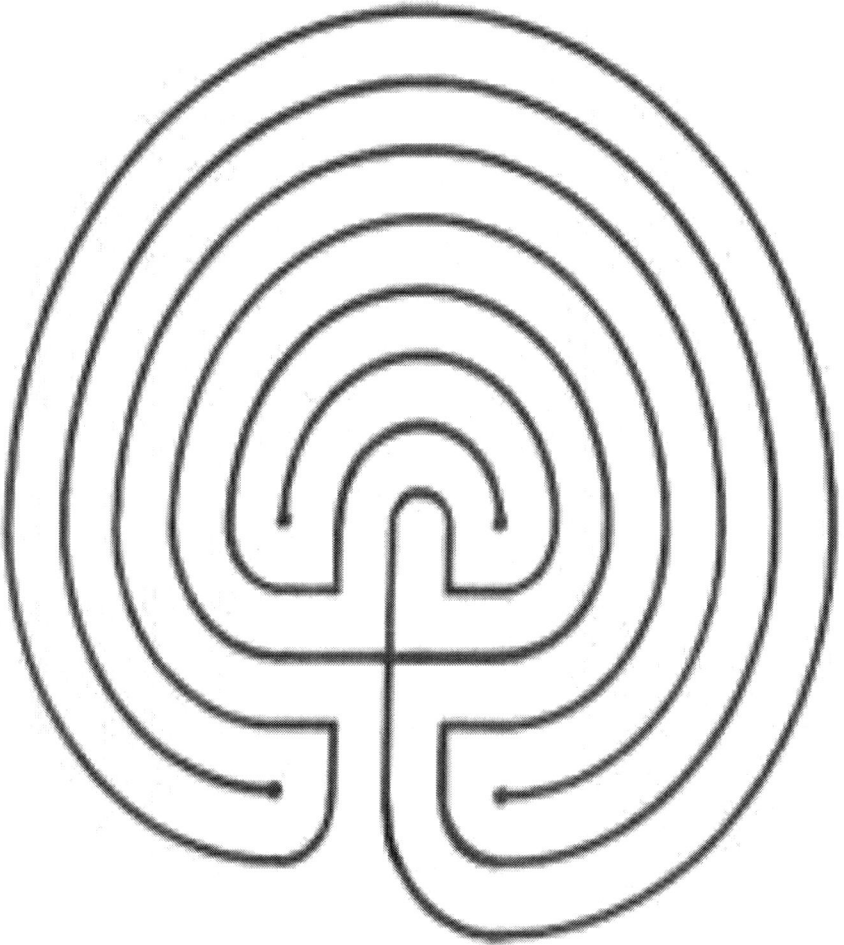

Labyrinth

Stand up right now! Bend over. How far can you reach without bending your legs? Rise back up and put your arms in the air. Wiggle those fingers. Slowly drop them to the side. Then up again! March in place to the count of 20. Jog in place for 30 seconds. Do this for ten minutes over and over again. Or just put on some music you love and MOVE for 10 minutes. Now, draw how you feel!

Draw!

Make a poster to motivate you or to remind you to exercise! Draw it below.

Draw!

Goal setting. What do you want to do next week for exercise? Map it out. Draw what you will do each day for at least 30 minutes. Be creative and share with others – who knows whom you might inspire?

MONDAY

TUESDAY

WEDNESDAY

THURSDAY

FRIDAY

THE WEEKEND . Plan something that involves moving your body. Where can you go and how will you move to improve your life? Draw a place and what you will do below.

Draw!

Chapter 10
Finances

Time is more valuable than money. You can get more money, but you cannot get more time.
    Jim Rohn

For I don't care too much for money, for money can't buy me love.
    The Beatles

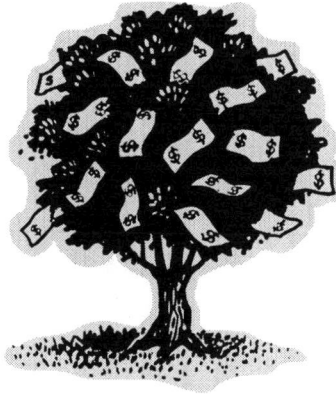

If you were fortunate enough to help contribute to your 401k, you might be doing well during your retirement, but, if like a lot of people, you don't have a lot of income to depend on, you may have to rethink what you want out of life.

As the two quotes remind us, life is not about money – it's about relationships, time, and love! But you are still going to have to pay the bills that come in regularly. Hopefully, you will not have a mortgage or rent to pay, but, if you do, try renegotiating for a lower interest rate. While you are doing that, try not to purchase big ticket items on time. Save up for those. I have found that not having to work keeps me spending less. There are actually days I stay home all day and don't buy a thing. Prioritize what you need and want. I'd rather give my kids small gifts of things they cannot afford. I love to spoil my granddaughter. But I don't need more clothing. I don't need more doodads in my house – chochtskys – you know those things that are everywhere and have to be dusted?

Keep busy with doing for others. It doesn't take a dime to meet a friend and walk and talk. It doesn't cost a cent to call a friend or go

over to visit. Church is a wonderful outlet for retirees. Join groups at your local church. Start new ones if there aren't any you think you'd like.

It's best to pay your bills online automatically. That way when you forget (and you will), they are paid and you are not stressed out. Invest a few hundred dollars a month and watch it grow. My investor Eric has done very well for me and I highly recommend starting a pension fund way before you actually retire (so if you are retired now, it isn't too late to save and earn more).

You have leisure time now so you can figure out where the least expensive gas is and you can go there. Of course, if it is twenty miles away, you might be cutting off your nose to spite your face....My local credit union offers all sorts of classes on retirement and spending and saving. I highly recommend you pay attention to these announcements and partake of the education.

And the best part is I can make money if I want. I can tutor kids @ $10 an hour and beat the heck out of a national tutoring company financially because I can meet the kids at the library and not pay the cost of an office....There are ways to exist comfortably. You just have to look for them.

Draw items you need to pay for, including your house. When you are finished, circle the ones that are the most difficult to pay....or the ones you are concerned with....

Draw!

Cut out of construction paper shapes to represent with whom you will be living during retirement. Are these people helping you with retirement financially?

Art Here!

Budget. Yes, you have to have a budget if you want to be less stressed. So, write your budget down and use colors to show what you are feeling about each item. Do you have enough at the end of the month? Enough money? Time? Sanity?

Write!

Sculpting! If you don't have any clay, you can make some wonderful clay – please look at the appendix and find the recipe. Now that you have returned from making a batch, take the clay and create anything you wish that might reflect your feelings about your financial status. What do you like/dislike about your piece?

Make some art!

Collaging! Find some magazines, the newspaper, and any loose photos you can – glue these below or on a larger sheet of paper. These can be things you want to buy, need to buy, or just have to buy – This will serve as a good visual reminder for you to save for these things! If you used a larger sheet of paper, write down below what you pasted on to the sheet of paper:

Write!

_____

_____

_____

_____

_____

_____

_____

_____

_____

Inside Out! Sometimes people think one thing about us and what we are really like on the inside is a whole different story. Find a large paper sack like the ones from the grocers. On the inside place photos, pictures, words, etc. that express how you really are. On the outside, decorate with pictures, words, etc. that describe how you believe others see you.

Make some art!

Chapter 11
Romance

Morris, an 82-year-old man, went to the doctor to get a physical.
A few days later the doctor saw Morris walking down the street with a gorgeous young lady on his arm.

A couple of days later, the doctor spoke to Morris and said, "You're really doing great, aren't you?" Morris replied, "Just doing what you said, Doctor, 'Get a hot mamma and be cheerful.'" The doctor said, "I didn't say that. I said you got a heart murmur and be careful."

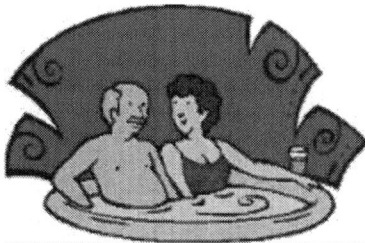

I can tell you as a veteran of marriage for over forty years, things just keep getting better, especially if they were okay in the beginning! Romance is still wonderful. I can't share our secrets or my hubby will get very mad, but that is a hint to one thing that has helped our marriage: respect. I respect his wishes and don't do things he would rather me not do, like sharing what he does and when he does it!

Talk to each other! That is so very important. Now that we are both retired and home, we do talk to each other and not only about the kids! We talk about the economy, schools, and enjoy watching the Science, Discover, and History channels, where we can learn new things and share with each other about them.

My sister is a widow and very, very tired of living alone. Her solution? To move when she retires to live next door to a dear friend of hers. She will have someone with whom to dialogue most of the time. Obviously, keeping busy helps keep one from getting lonely.

I noticed there are many dating agencies and some that are just for seniors. You can meet others for socialization and even romance, if you so desire. Why not go down to the local senior center? Each one has its own particular flavor. If you don't like one, then go visit another. Some churches have social groups for seniors. Check them out! You don't have to go back if you don't like it.

Keep up your sense of humor. That is the #1 ticket to romance. Be able to laugh off things. And, ladies, this is for you: don't try to change that man. Be realistic. If you've been around him a while, you know what he is like. If he never picked up his dishes, or helped around the house, why in the world would you think he would start now? Same thing for the guys – if she has been doing all the cooking for years, why do you think she might like your suggestions in the kitchen now?

Talk to each other. Find out what the other person wants and/or needs. You might be surprised that you can even be happier than you are. The most romantic moment this year was....ah, shucks, remember I can't tell ya? But, believe me, it cost nothing and was worth a million!

Self Portrait: Draw what you think you look like. Take your time. Look in a mirror. Just draw the lines and contours of your face. You will see one of me in the appendix. Yes, it was shocking to see all the lines and contours, but after a while, I decided it doesn't matter – I am wild and crazy on the outside and still 16, although I don't look that way in the mirror!

Draw!

List by drawing five places, events, or gifts that were memorable to you – perhaps, we can say, even romantic?

Write!

_____

_____

_____

_____

_____

_____

_____

_____

_____

Why do you think these were romantic? Are they self-explanatory?

Draw!

DRAW the ideal man/woman of your choice! No holds barred! Just have fun with this assignment. What are the characteristics that this person has that appeal to you? I use a template called *THE MAN* and write qualities on each of these areas:

Head (what does s/he think)

Eyes (what s/he sees)

Nose (favorite fragrances)

Mouth (type of speech that person has or uses)

Shoulders (can you lean on his/her shoulder?)

Heart (what does that person feel?)

Hands (what does that person do with his/her hands?)

Feet (where does that person like to go?). Have fun with this one! You might use a larger sheet of paper, if you'd like! Add hair and clothing to complete your ideal mate!

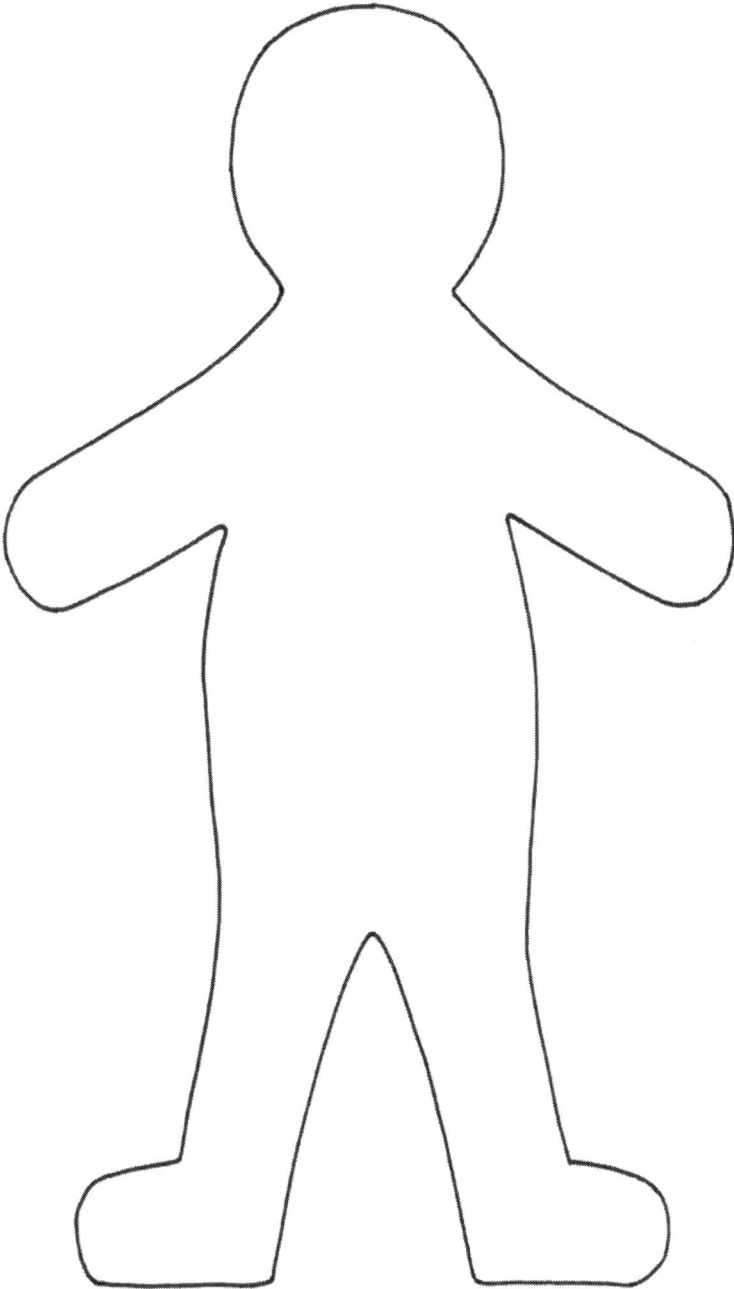

Write or Post and AD! Have fun with this one! Write an ad for yourself! What are your good points? Your selling points, so to speak?

Chapter 12
Five Senses

All we have to believe with is our senses, the tools we use to perceive the world: our sight, our touch, our memory. If they lie to us, then nothing can be trusted. And even if we do not believe, then still we cannot travel in any other way than the road our senses show us; and we must walk that road to the end.

Neil Gaiman

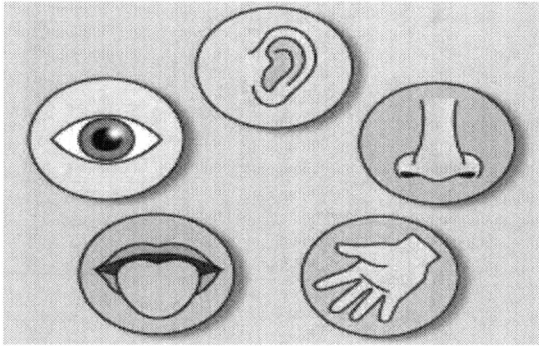

Using your five senses seems like a no-brainer. But think of the last time you used your sense of smell other than to notify you that the kitchen was on fire. When was the last time you brought in great smelling flowers or just sprayed on some lavender upon your bed linens? Integrating all the senses into your daily life is a way to lift your spirits, as well as create new sensorial memories. Serving piping hot and spicy warm apple pancakes and presenting them with panache is what makes breakfast special, or even dinner, if you decide to serve them then!

Listening to a variety of music is like taking an extra pill of happiness in the morning! Broaden your scope of listening music. I love Pandora, which I get for FREE on the Internet. I type in a song or an artist and I get an amazing tailored-for-me music station. Some days I'm in a mood for rock and roll of the 60's but other times I need to listen to Enya. The world is your music store!

Movement is very important for our joints and wellbeing. Turn up Pandora and sway to the music in your nightgown or your shorts. You don't have to go somewhere to dance! Exercise to the music. As long as you are moving you are healing your body and mind.

Use your hands to create. Craft projects, building projects, redesigning your furniture layout in the living room – all these create a phenomena called positive movement. PM works best when you regularly perform movement actions that are out of the norm for you.

The ideal for us might be to dance in the rose gardens, with the rain gently falling upon us, as we taste the drops descending upon us.....yes, all our senses need to be stimulated in order to create the best living environment. Ensure that you have enough sunlight – seeing the brightness of day, feeling the heat rays, walking slowly, listening to the birds chirp. How can it get better than that?

Draw something you can do that uses all your senses!
Dream! Something you haven't done before?

Write!

_____

_____

_____

_____

_____

_____

_____

_____

_____

_____

_____

Draw!

Collage! Find some places you might want to visit. How could you use all five of your senses in this new adventure?

Make some art!

DRUMMING! Try beating out the rhythm to a favorite song on the radio. Try a different surface to drum on. Note the aromas around you – is it a fresh crisp autumn air or the warm blades of grass type of smell you notice? Stop what do you hear? Can you feel the beat of your heart? Draw what you feel....

Draw!

Make Your own play dough! New recipe!

2 cups flour
2 cups warm water
1 cup salt
2 Tablespoons vegetable oil
1 Tablespoon cream of tartar (optional for improved elasticity)

food coloring (liquid, powder, or unsweetened drink mix)
scented oils
Mix all of the ingredients together, and stir over low heat. The dough will begin to thicken until it resembles mashed potatoes.

When the dough pulls away from the sides and clumps in the center, as shown below, remove the pan from heat and allow the dough to cool enough to handle. Turn the dough out onto a clean counter or silicone mat, and knead vigorously until it becomes silky-smooth. Divide the dough into balls for coloring.

Make a hole in the center of the ball, and drop in some food coloring. Fold the dough over, working the food color through the body of the play dough, trying to keep the raw dye away from your hands and the counter. You could use gloves or plastic wrap at this stage to keep your hands clean-only the concentrated dye will color your skin, so as soon as it's worked in, bare hands are fine.

Play and store

WRITE YOUR REACTIONS HERE: **SMELL SIGHT TOUCH SOUNDS TASTE** (not recommended!)

Write!

_____

_____

_____

_____

_____

_____

_____

_____

IMPROVE your sense of smell! Do the following:
- ✓ Breathe deeper whenever you have a chance.
- ✓ Fix allergies.
- ✓ Stop and smell the "roses."
- ✓ Try various scents at the perfume counter.
- ✓ Notice the air about you outside – what do you smell?

DRAW YOUR NOSE!

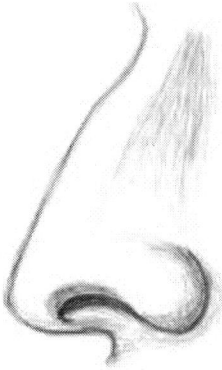

IMPROVE your sight by following these suggestions:
- ✓ Make sure your eyes are moist (either cry or use drops!)
- ✓ Try looking around in a dark room.
- ✓ Stare up at the sky – (don't look at the sun, however)
- ✓ Look to the side of you (using your peripheral vision).
- ✓ Wear sunglasses only when it's too bright outside!

DRAW YOUR EYES!

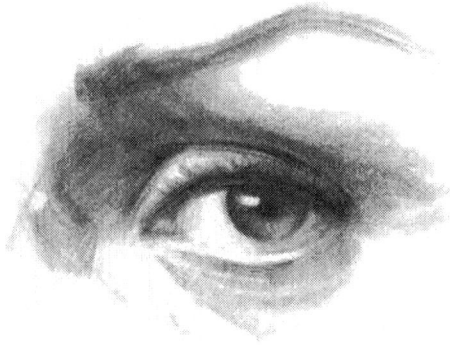

IMPROVE your sense of touch by practicing these:
- ✓ Touch a variety of fabrics. Note the differences.
- ✓ Exercise your hands by gripping a squeeze ball.
- ✓ Touch a variety of hot, warm, cold, and cool items. Notice how they each feel.
- ✓ Run your hands through your hair!
- ✓ Pick a variety of stones up – feel each one. Rough? Smooth?

TRACE YOUR HAND! Left or right – your call!

IMPROVE your sense of hearing. We can all use a bit of help here!

- ✓ Listen to a variety of music.
- ✓ Keep volumes low so you can really attend.
- ✓ Listen to the sounds of nature.
- ✓ As you sit in a waiting room, notice the variety of sounds.
- ✓ Truly listen to others. What are they saying?

DRAW YOUR EAR!

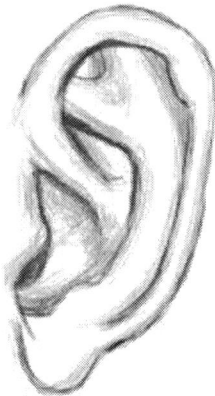

Chapter 13
Defying the Odds

There were people who went to sleep last night, poor and rich and white and black, but they will never wake again. And those dead folks would give anything at all for just five minutes of this weather or ten minutes of plowing. So you watch yourself about complaining. What you're supposed to do when you don't like a thing is change it. If you can't change it, change the way you think about it."
— Maya Angelou

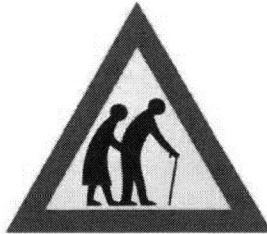

Something phenomenal that I've learned in my later years is that your reality is exactly that – reality! For instance, when the daughter in law says that she is too busy to see you the next week, make that your reality. She is too busy, and then get on with life. You could try to understand and see through that phrase. Is she really too busy? Too busy because she doesn't want to see us? Or is she mad? Just take it for what it is. It is what it is. That is my new mantra. Hard to teach someone ensconced in WHYs all the time to just accept and get along with life. But it can work. And, boy, will you ever be happier for it.

Learn to be in the moment! When you finally achieve this, you will find that you are happier and more satisfied with life in general. Being in the moment means relishing what is. Not asking what could be or worrying about the future....

A friend recently made an astute statement. Perhaps the reason generations do not seem to connect is that the older generation are living in the past and the younger generation are living in the future. If they both lived in the moment, perhaps they'd be at the same place at the same time. It makes sense. That does not mean we shouldn't deal with the past or future, but it does mean we should not live in those spaces.

Create new memories. Try out something new. We're trying to figure out if we really want to go to a Tree House B&B. Zip line? Horseback riding? Maybe not, but the tree house itself sounds kind of fun....Get excited about something in life and enjoy that something.

Or travel somewhere you've never been before. Change up the route you come home from church. Go another way home. Keep those neurons firing and the engines running smoothly!

Draw a tree house you might rent for a few days. What would you put in it? Where would it be? Have fun with this one!

Draw!

Collage with some clip art from Google. Mountains?
Lakes? Boats? Space? Cut and paste those below.
Which are your favorites? Which might you truly try?

Make some art!

Brainstorm something you've never done before.
Draw them below.
Circle the ones you may want to try.

Write!

_____

_____

_____

_____

_____

_____

_____

_____

_____

Draw!

Dream Big! It can't hurt and certainly might provide a few minutes of fun. Draw things you once wanted to do and just never got around to....still wanna do them? Why or why not? Talk first, then draw!

Write!

_____

_____

_____

_____

_____

_____

_____

_____

_____

_____

_____

Draw!

CHOOSE one of your craziest ideas and explore the possibilities by drawing a web and writing pros and cons. Example:

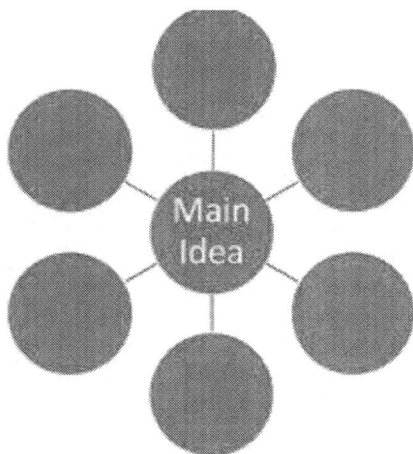

LEARN something new and prosper! Think about something you want to know more about. Write it down or draw it. Research it and put your results below. Drawing is a fine way, but you can collage with photos, clip art, etc.

Write!

_____

_____

_____

_____

_____

_____

_____

_____

_____

_____

Draw!

Chapter 14
Write Your Own Story

*An **autobiography** usually reveals nothing bad about its writer except his memory.*
Benjamin Franklin

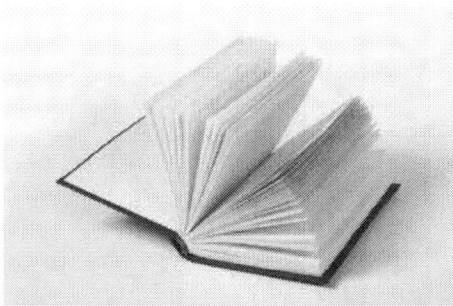

No one would have believed it that I would retire and write and publish three books, with two more on the horizon. What is it about us that makes us want to share our diatribe with others? It boils down to the inner desire to make a difference, to share our talents, albeit meager at times, with the world to come, as it were. I have several family members who are actually much better writers than I. What is the difference between them and me? I do it. They don't. They write, read, reread, and toss their work. They are never satisfied with it. I, on the other hand, probably have lower standards than they (I'm sure they would agree), but I have learned that I will never be perfect and I do the best I am able....

So, look at your life. What is your story? Perhaps it is a compilation of things or maybe it's something conjured up in your head. With the advent of various sites that publish on demand, you can create something fairly inexpensively to share with your family. One of my recent books is a summary of all the things I learned in and out of graduate school that pertains to teaching reading. I gave a copy to my three-year old granddaughter. Surely she won't be reading it for a long time, if ever. But I can guarantee you she will keep it, for her picture at 18 months is on the cover – she is reading a book and the chances are that book might even make it to show and tell one day. What a legacy for that child!

Several publishers provide a workbook style for you to fill in answers to questions. That might be the lazy man's way of doing it, but think about your particular story. Perhaps you have photos you could scan and describe, making an enjoyable photo book. Some of you have had amazing experiences. Describe them. Draw about them. Share them on paper and give them as gifts to your family.

Start by thinking about writing and brainstorming. Several ways work well in order to stimulate your writing. As a former English teacher, I was able to even get the most turned off and tuned out 8th grade boys to write, so I know you can do it!

Close your eyes and think of your life. Perhaps your family would be interested in what it was like as a teen in the 60's or 50's....what would you share with them? Remember to keep from telling – but show with your words. Use descriptive words – talk about the colors, smells, and shapes.

BRAINSTORM! You can make your own, but this is a start! Fill it out with information you think you can write about....

Write!

_____

_____

_____

_____

_____

_____

_____

_____

_____

_____

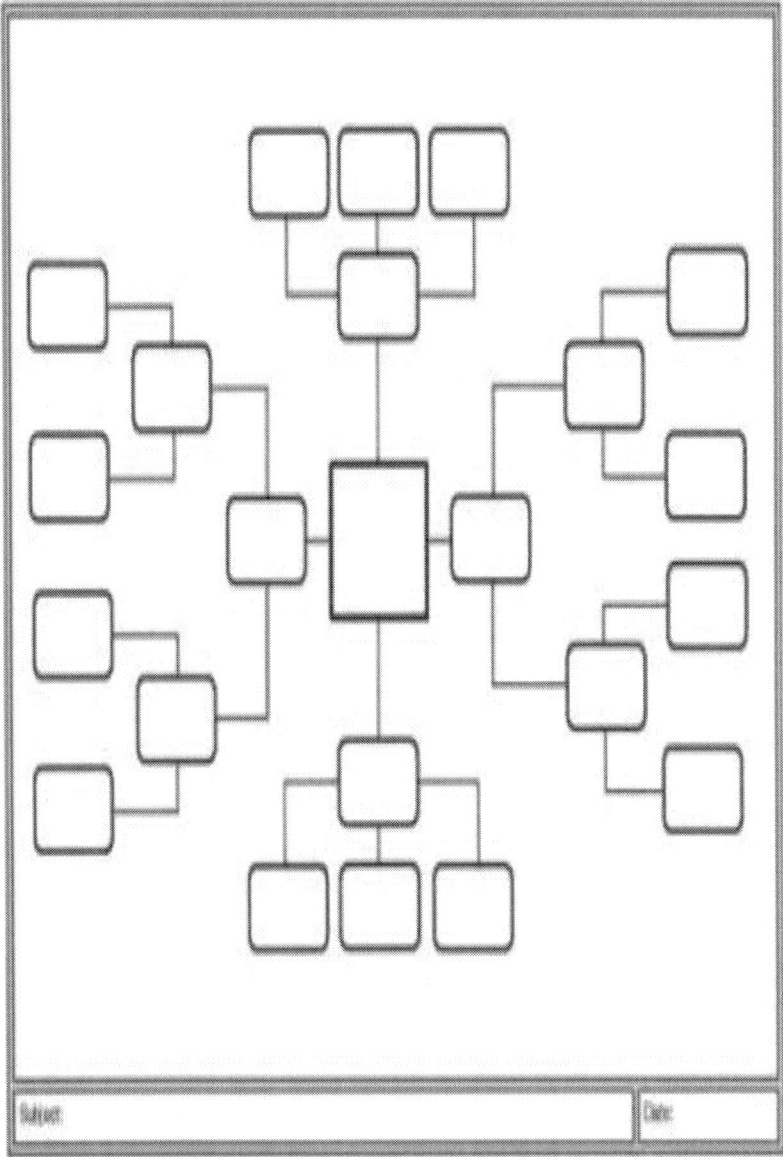

Subject: Date:

FOCUS on one subject. For instance, the 60's. Where were you? What did you do? What thoughts did you have? Your icons? Your heroes? Your activities? Draw them randomly here. Which ones make you smile? Circle those!

Write!

_____

_____

_____

_____

_____

_____

_____

_____

_____

Draw!

DO NOT TELL EVERY DETAIL! Pick out an era that was interesting to you and share that short story. You don't have to write a novel. Just share some part of you. Draw what that story might look like.

Write!

_____

_____

_____

_____

_____

_____

_____

_____

_____

Draw!

Fantasize! What could have been? Should have been? Might have been? What could never be? Should never be? Won't ever be? Draw those! Have fun with this one....

Write!

_____

_____

_____

_____

_____

_____

_____

_____

_____

_____

Draw!

Title your story....If your story were a movie, what would it be called? Make a flyer for that movie below.

Draw!

Characters. Draw the main characters in your life story. Draw them so we have an idea of who they really are...what they really did....and what they really might say.....

Write!

_____

_____

_____

_____

_____

_____

_____

_____

_____

_____

Vignettes. Can't write a whole book? Just write some fun things that have happened to you – or memorable events. They don't have to be connected! Add photos!

Write!

_____

_____

_____

_____

_____

_____

_____

_____

_____

_____

_____

Draw!

Chapter 15
Don't Depend on Your Kids!

*We need to restore the full meaning of that
old word, duty. It is the other side of rights.*
~Pearl Buck

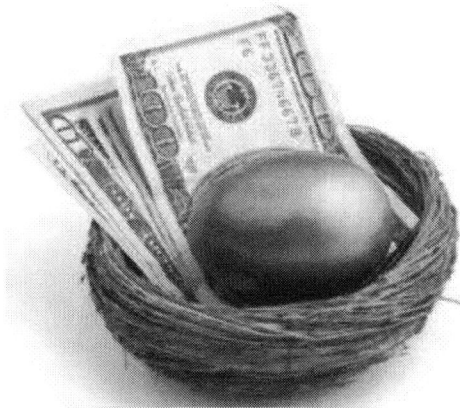

Your children have a life of their own to live and it does not include you on a daily basis. That is fact. Maybe there are exceptions, but I do not know of many. This was one of the hardest things to do as I entered "empty nest" syndrome. Why, I needed to see and talk to my grown sons every day, uh, I mean every week. And then they got married and their wives did not appreciate my clinginess. I did not see it as clinginess, but I suppose it was, depending on one's perspective. Not working anymore, I had way lots of time to spend and usually spent it harassing the kids. Okay, I think if I had a daughter it would be different, but I have given birth to and raised three men. I need to fade into the background and be there for them. That's hard to do.

Find things to do and things that occupy your time. Write, draw, visit others, and read. Do what makes you feel happy. We baby boomers are an awesome lot. We are vibrant and educated for the most part. We can still be a vital part of society.

Walk dogs – talk to others. Visit the local coffee shop. Travel! Compliment others. Make life worth living. You won't be as depressed and you may even be more fulfilled than ever!

Take a deep breath, wrap your arms around yourself, and feel the love!

KIDS? OR NO KIDS? Even if you don't have kids, there are people you will start wanting to engage with more. Before you overwhelm them, check out why you are getting in touch....Draw some of the reasons you might start "bugging" someone....

Relax! Draw some things you like to do below.

Write!

_____

_____

_____

_____

_____

_____

_____

_____

_____

_____

_____

_____

Draw!

When you get the urge to call that person for the umpteenth time again, try doing one of these activities.

Play hangman! Forgot how?

— — — — — — — — — —

1. Play individually or in groups.
2. Select a letter of the alphabet.
3. If the letter is contained in the word/phrase, the group or individual takes another turn guessing a letter
4. If the letter is not contained in the word/phrase, a portion of the hangman is added.
5. The game continues until:
   1. the word/phrase is guessed (all letters are revealed) – WINNER or,
   2. all the parts of the hangman are displayed – LOSER

answer: retirement

Cut Construction Family: Take construction paper and create shapes for those you consider family. Place them below. Look at how they are placed. What can you read into that?

Make some art!

Write!

_____

_____

_____

_____

_____

_____

_____

_____

_____

_____

_____

_____

Look at both sides! Complete the other side of a photo from a magazine or newspaper. Cut out the photo and fold it vertically. Glue half here and then recreate the other side. Remember, everything has two sides....)

Make some art!

Write!

_____

_____

_____

_____

_____

_____

_____

_____

_____

_____

_____

_____

Appendix
Resources you may enjoy...

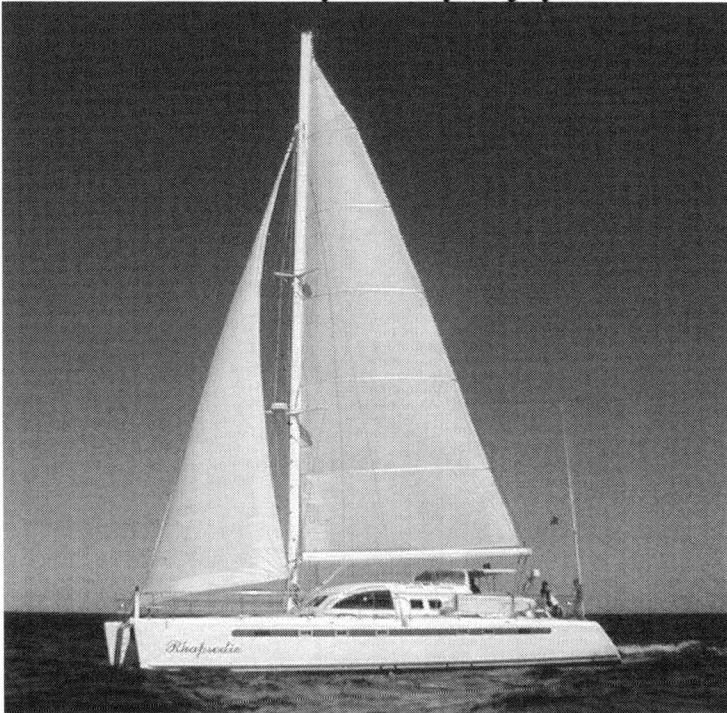

Elder treks-This is a truly outstanding tour company that specializes in senior citizens and single seniors. They offer exciting trips all over the world at reasonable prices. They have a huge variety of domestic travel opportunities. They offer luxury and value. Plus they give you personalized care with small tour groups. I cannot say enough good things about this tour company. They have a fantastic reputation which speaks for itself. Please visit their website to see what they offer in domestic travel.
http://www.eldertreks.com/

Smithsonian Education Tours - This is a very unique tour company because they offer trips that also teach you something. You are truly never too old to learn something new and this tour company is willing to teach as they travel you around. They have many lovely trips in the United States to interest any traveler. Please visit their website for more information.
http://www.smithsonianjourneys.org/?src

Here is a wonderful senior travel site that offer advice to seniors who are considering planning that once in a

lifetime trip. There is a lot of information on this website to help seniors in every aspect of trip planning.
http://www.tripconnect.com/tripconnect/Seniors

This is another senior travel help site that offers advice and information on traveling in your golden years.
http://www.suddenlysenior.com/TRAVELPAGE.html

This is another site that helps seniors with travel advice. It also helps the single senior plan a trip and save money. http://www.catholicseniors.com/time-to-travel.html

Collette Vacations - This is a company that has been in business for many years. It has gained an outstanding reputation for offering deluxe tours at reasonable prices. Their prices range from as little as $700 per person on up. They travel through all the states and they offer luxury motor coach travel with knowledgeable tour guides. They try to keep the groups small. Normally they range from 16-24 people per trip. Please visit their website for more information on their wonderful travel in the United States. You can also order a free brochure from them

that lists all their tours and prices.
http://www.collettevacations.com/

Learn about living more simply and fully:
http://zenhabits.net/simple-living-manifesto-72-ideas-to-simplify-your-life/

Mandalas are seen in nature. They represent the stars, the earth, the heavenly bodies, a person's face, the iris of the eye, and all throughout nature you will see mandalas.
http://www.abgoodwin.com/mandala/ccweb.shtml

Learning more about labyrinths:
http://www.lessons4living.com/labyrinth.htm

To find a labyrinth in your area, check out
http://labyrinthlocator.com/.

More than you'd ever want to know about finances, investing, etc.:
http://www.sec.gov/investor/seniors.shtml

Learning from others about finances:
http://www.pickthebrain.com/blog/10-inspirational-quotes-to-apply-to-your-finances/

Recipe for homemade clay:
HOMEMADE MODELING CLAY

2 c. baking soda
1 1/4 c. water
1 c. cornstarch
Mix cornstarch and soda, then add water and
mix thoroughly. Bring to a boil, stirring
constantly. Thicken to consistency of mashed
potatoes. Let it cool just enough to handle, then
form into desired shapes. Unused portions will
not keep long, but tightly covered will keep
enough to make holiday decorations, etc. Let
dry completely (at least 36 hours). Color with
paint or felt tip markers or coat with shellac or
clear nail polish. You can even make jewelry!

Helping seniors website:
http://www.seniorark.com/senior_tips_money.htm

Government website for helping seniors:
http://www.usa.gov/Topics/Seniors.shtml

Humor site for seniors:
http://www.swapmeetdave.com/Humor/Seniors.htm

Cathy's art therapy site is very helpful – check it out!
http://www.cathymalchiodi.com/

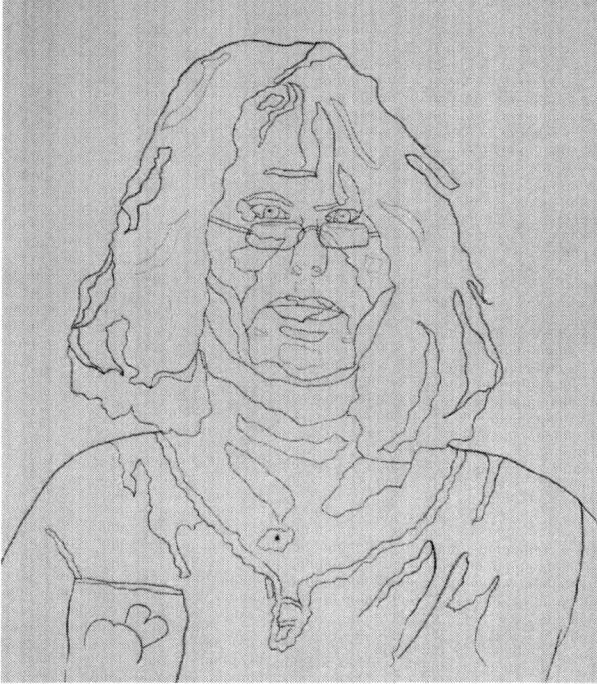

Contour drawing:

Just look in the mirror and draw lines where you see darker and lighter areas.

http://drawsketch.about.com/cs/drawinglessons/a/contourdrawing.htm

http://en.wikipedia.org/wiki/Blind_contour_drawing

Vacation in a tree house!
http://www.treehouses.com/

Play games online! Good for your brain and outlook on life. http://games.aarp.org/games/crossword-easy.aspx

http://www.learn-to-draw-right.com/right-brain-left-brain.html Great for mental stimulation and fun.

Introduction to Art as Therapy and Art Therapy

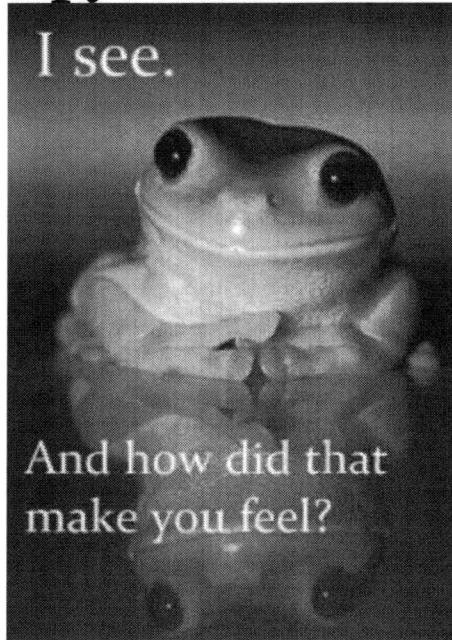

I see.

And how did that make you feel?

Art as Therapy

Doing art is therapeutic. You do not have to have an art therapist to guide you to benefit from art as therapy. Any kind of gardening, creating, art, etc. is great for your mind and soul. The process is wonderful and it doesn't matter if you have a great product at the end. Just enjoy and live!

Art Therapy (Psychotherapy)

According to the **'What is Art Therapy?'** brochure from the website of (BAAT - British Association of Art Therapists),

"Art therapy is a form of psychotherapy that uses art media as its primary mode of communication. It is practiced by qualified, registered Art Therapists who work with children, young people, adults and the elderly.

Clients who can use art therapy may have a wide range of difficulties, disabilities or diagnoses. These include, for example, emotional, behavioral or mental health problems, learning or physical disabilities, life-limiting conditions, brain-injury or neurological conditions and physical illness. Art therapy may be provided for groups, or for individuals, depending on clients' needs. It is not a recreational activity or an art lesson, although the sessions can be enjoyable. Clients do not need to have any previous experience or expertise in art."

The American Art Therapy Association describes it this way:

"Art therapy is the therapeutic use of art making, within a professional relationship, by people who experience illness, trauma or challenges in living, and by people who seek personal development. Through creating art and reflecting on the art products and processes, people can increase awareness of self and others cope with symptoms, stress and traumatic experiences; enhance cognitive abilities; and enjoy the life-affirming pleasures of making art.

"Art therapy is a mental health profession that uses the creative process of art making to improve and enhance the physical, mental and emotional well-being of individuals of all ages. It is based on the belief that the creative process involved in artistic self-expression

214

helps people to resolve conflicts and problems, develop interpersonal skills, manage behavior, reduce stress, increase self-esteem and self-awareness, and achieve insight. Art therapy integrates the fields of human development, visual art (drawing, painting, sculpture, and other art forms), and the creative process with models of counseling and psychotherapy."

DISCLAIMER

This book is not written to be art therapy, but, rather, as art AS therapy. If it were truly art therapy, I would be there with you, changing the directives, thoughtfully guiding you, and delivering psychotherapy. I am not there. You are not with an art therapist and you are using the book to relax and understand yourself. You are doing art AS therapy.

☺ *lola*

Notes and Doodles
Use the next few pages for your notes, additions, questions, and photos. Enjoy and please share your responses with us @ masabitherapist@gmail.com

Art As Therapy for Retirees

Art As Therapy for Retirees

221

Art As Therapy for Retirees

Art As Therapy for Retirees

Art As Therapy for Retirees

Art As Therapy for Retirees

Made in the USA
Charleston, SC
18 December 2012